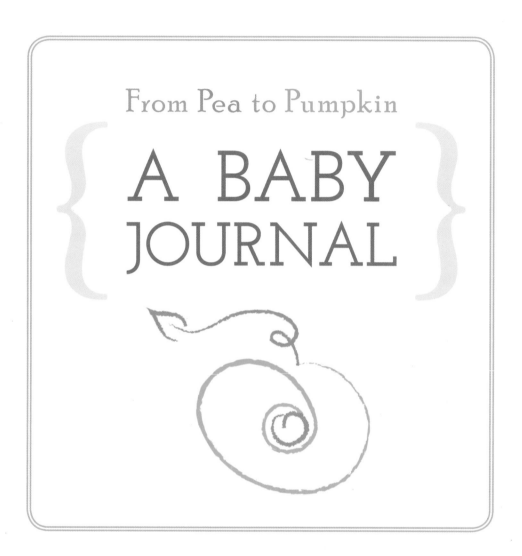

From Pea to Pumpkin

{ A BABY JOURNAL }

GERALYN BRODER MURRAY

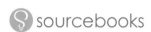

For my no longer babies but my forever loves:
Reese and Finn.
And for Chris, as always.

This publication is designed to provide accurate and authoritative information in regard to the subject matter covered. It is sold with the understanding that the publisher is not engaged in rendering legal, accounting, or other professional service. If legal advice or other expert assistance is required, the services of a competent professional person should be sought. —From a Declaration of Principles Jointly Adopted by a Committee of the American Bar Association and a Committee of Publishers and Associations

All brand names and product names used in this book are trademarks, registered trademarks, or trade names of their respective holders. Sourcebooks, Inc. is not associated with any product or vendor in this book.

Published by Sourcebooks, Inc.
P.O. Box 4410, Naperville, Illinois 60567-4410
(630) 961-3900
Fax: (630) 961-2168
www.sourcebooks.com

Printed and bound in China.
OGP 10 9 8 7 6 5

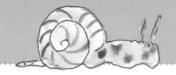

This baby journal is for

_____

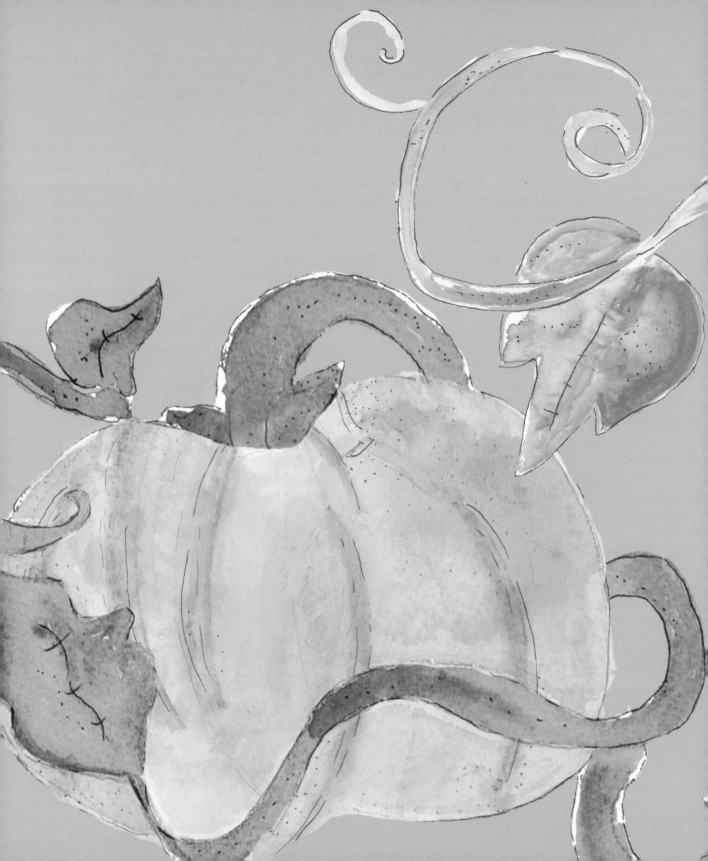

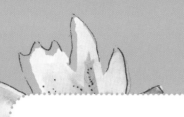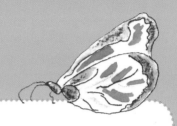

Dear Baby,

Someone who loves you bought this sweet little journal to help remember how tiny you once were, way back in the very beginning. One day you will walk and talk and leave Legos all over the house and play your very first T-ball game and refuse to eat anything but mac and cheese for dinner for three weeks straight, and the people who love you will barely be able to remember (or believe!) that you once only slept and ate and pooped. They might not remember the name of the doctor who delivered you or when you first rolled over or whether your first word was "dog" or "bagel." This little journal will remind them of all of that; one day they will pick up this book (or you will) and all the dozens of special baby moments from your first year will be there for the remembering, for the reliving, for the storytelling. Someone bought this journal because you, sweet baby, are already so loved and no one ever wants to forget a single thing about how you made your family, a family.

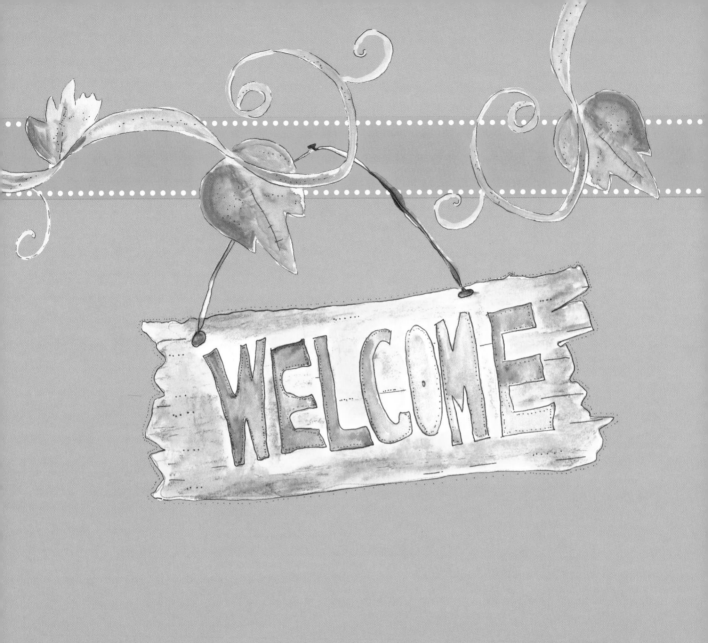

Look who sprouted!

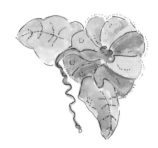

Place photo here.

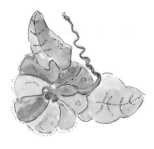

The world is so lucky to have you.

Your name: _____.

Parents' names: _____

_____

_____.

Born on: _____

at _____

_____.

Time: _____

_____.

Weight: _____

_____.

Length: _____

_____.

Delivered by: _____

A bit about your birth: _____

_____

_____

_____

_____

_____.

The Story of Your Name

Why we chose this name for you: _____

_____

_____

_____

_____

_____

_____

_____

_____

_____

_____

_____ .

How we discovered your name: _____

_____

_____ .

What it means: _____

_____

_____

_____

Other names on our list: _____

_____

_____

_____

Place baby announcement here.

The Story of Your Arrival

We first knew you were really coming when _____
_____.

It took _____ for you to get here.

We _____
_____ while we waited for you.

You were born at _____
_____, with
_____ right there waiting for you.

The first thing we thought when you arrived was _____
_____
_____.

We thought you looked _____
_____ and a lot like
_____.

The first few people who came to see you were _____
_____
_____.

We couldn't be more happy / relieved / exhausted /
hungry / giddy / emotional / grateful.

(Circle what applies.)

First Family Photo

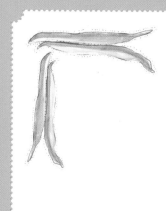

Place photo here.

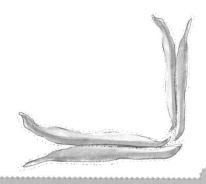

Letter from Your Family on Your Day of Birth

Your Home

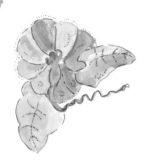

Place photo here.

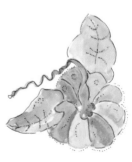

Your first address: _____

_____

_____

_____.

It took _____ minutes to get you home safely. You wore

_____

_____

_____

_____ for the occasion.

The first thing you did at home was _____

_____

_____

_____

_____.

The first thing we did was _____

_____

_____

_____

_____.

We couldn't be more happy / relieved / exhausted /
hungry / giddy / emotional / grateful.

(Circle what applies.)

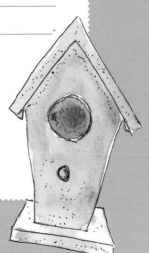

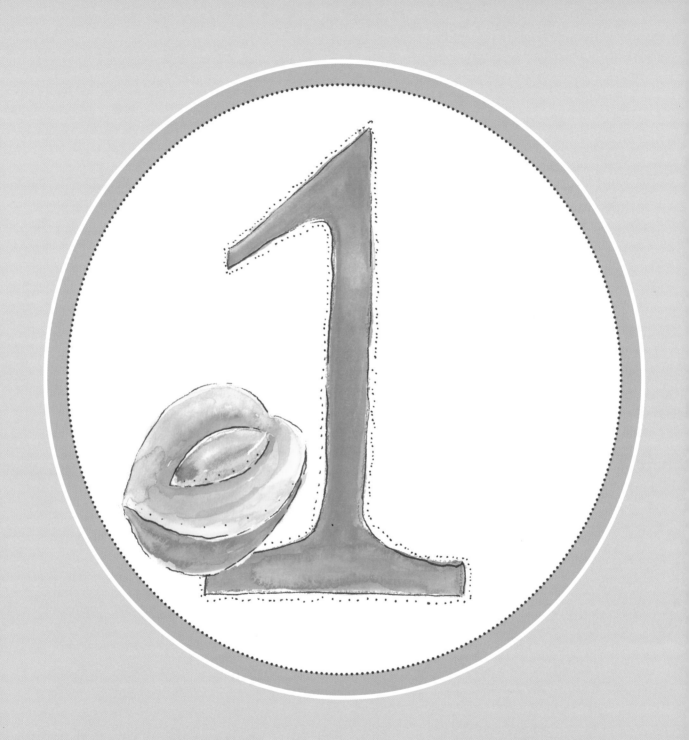

MONTH

You are a little peach.

Place photo here.

Height: _____

Weight: _____

Thoughts about Month One

_____

_____

_____

_____

_____

_____

_____

_____

_____

_____

_____

_____

_____

_____

_____

_____

_____

_____

_____

_____

ONE MONTH

The first week was _____

_____.

The people who helped included _____

_____

_____.

Thank goodness for _____

_____.

How/if/when you slept, it was _____

_____.

We comforted you by _____

_____

_____.

We are already in love with your _____

_____.

What we don't want to forget about this month of your life is _____

_____

_____.

We couldn't be more happy / relieved / exhausted /
hungry / giddy / emotional / grateful.

(Circle what applies.)

Little hands. Big heart.

Place drawing, photo, or handprint of baby's hands here.

Little feet. Big love.

Place drawing, photo, or footprint of baby's feet here.

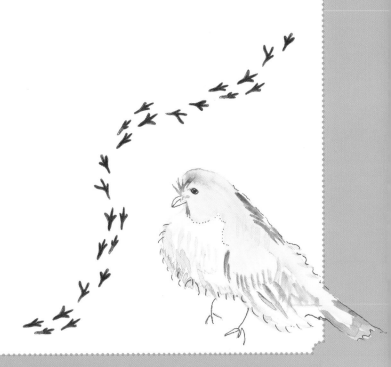

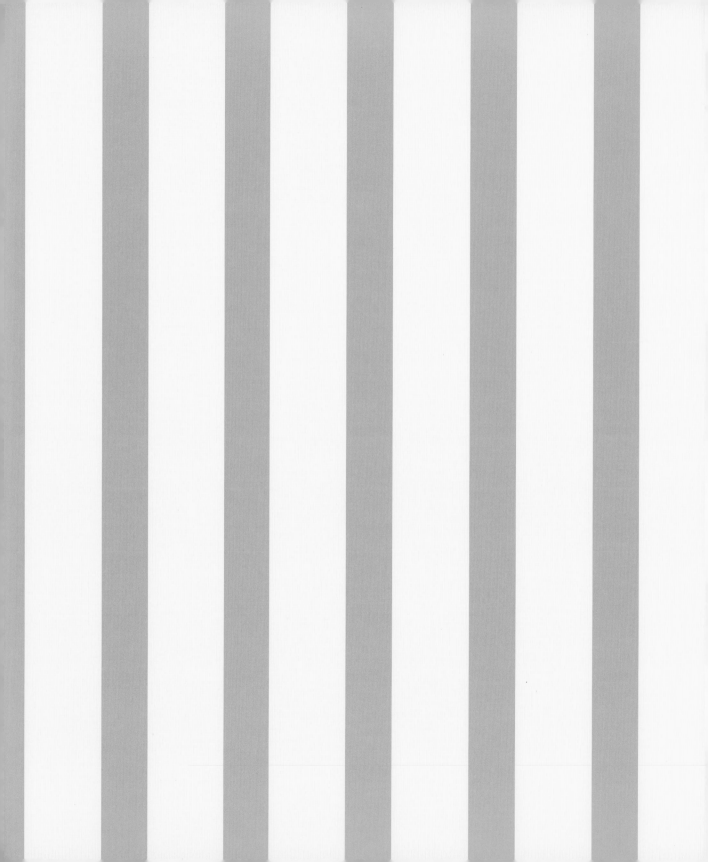

Pumpkin Pie Chart

Baby's day on: _____

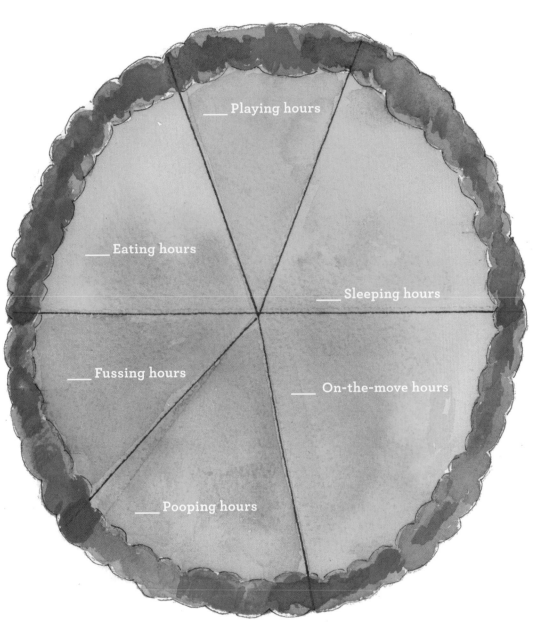

___ Playing hours

___ Eating hours

___ Sleeping hours

___ Fussing hours

___ On-the-move hours

___ Pooping hours

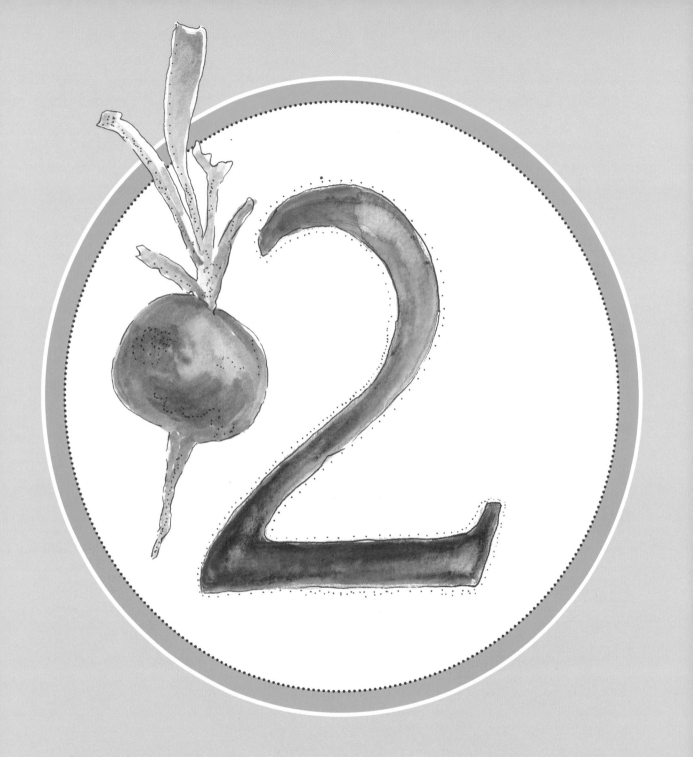

MONTHS

What a sweet baby.

Place photo here.

Height: _____

Weight: _____

Thoughts about Month Two

_____

_____

_____

_____

_____

_____

_____

_____

_____

_____

_____

_____

_____

_____

_____

_____

_____

_____

TWO MONTHS

We can't stop looking at your _____

_____

_____.

The sounds you respond to the most are _____

_____

_____.

What you seem to love best right now is _____

_____

_____.

Your personality is starting to shine through and it looks like this:

_____

_____

_____

_____.

What we don't want to forget about this month of your life is _____

_____

_____.

We couldn't be more happy / relieved / exhausted /
hungry / giddy / emotional / grateful.

(Circle what applies.)

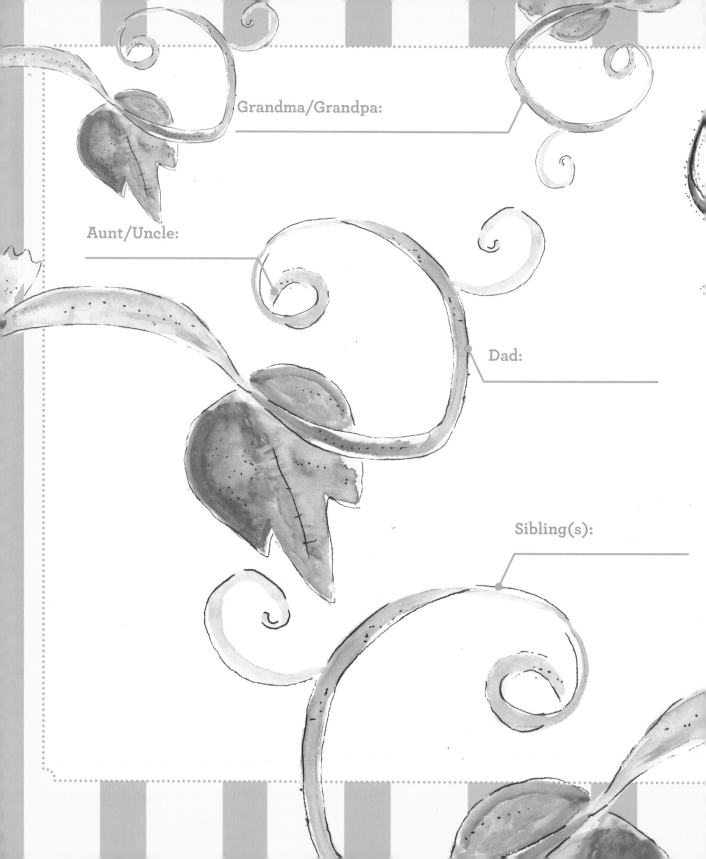

Grandma/Grandpa:

Aunt/Uncle:

Dad:

Sibling(s):

Family Vine

Grandma/Grandpa:

Mom:

Baby:

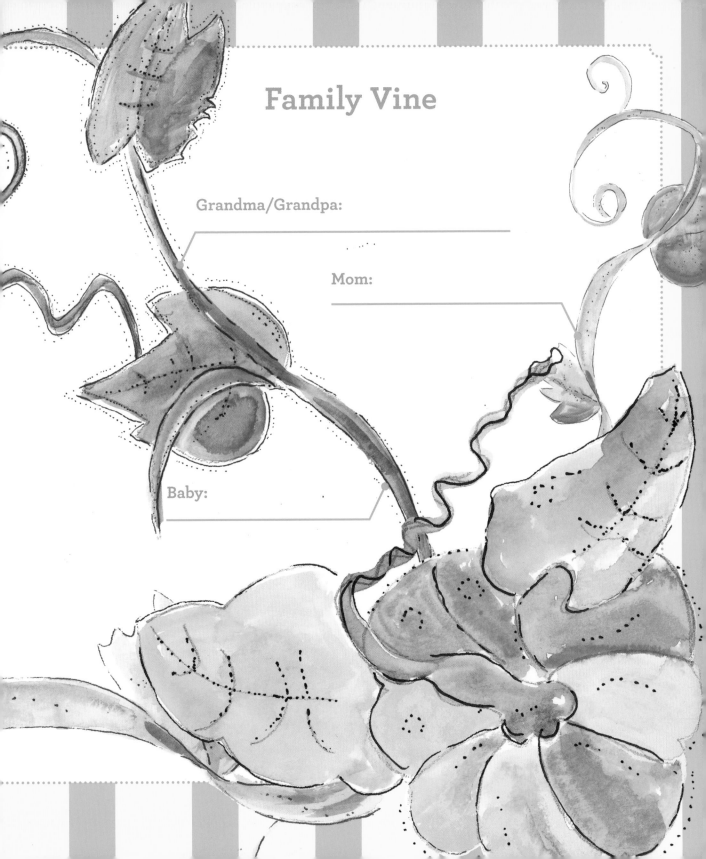

Someone Special and You

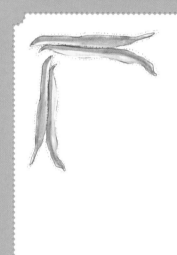

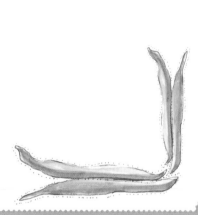

Place photo here.

You Are Very Popular

Your guest list:

1. _____

2. _____

3. _____

4. _____

5. _____

6. _____

7. _____

8. _____

9. _____

10. _____

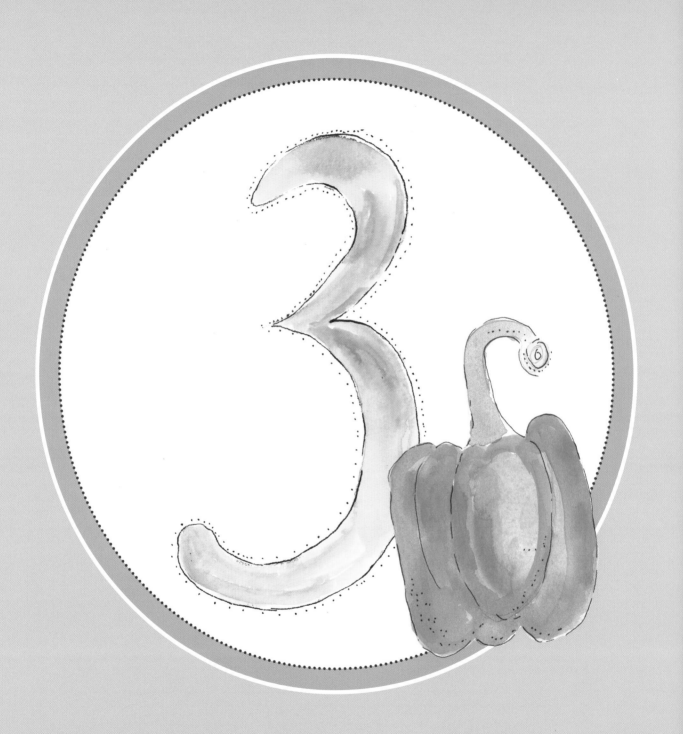

MONTHS

You are a cutie patootie.

Place photo here.

Height: _____

Weight: _____

Thoughts about Month Three

_____

_____

_____

_____

_____

_____

_____

_____

_____

_____

_____

_____

_____

_____

_____

_____

_____

THREE MONTHS

Supposedly, you are on a schedule right now. It looks like this:

_____

_____.

Right now, you look a lot like _____

_____.

And maybe _____ too.

Your favorite thing to do seems to be _____

_____.

Your smile is _____

_____.

Our nights pretty much consist of _____

_____.

What we want you to know about your family right now is _____

_____.

What we don't want to forget about this month of your life is _____

_____

_____.

We couldn't be more happy / relieved / exhausted /
hungry / giddy / emotional / grateful.

(Circle what applies.)

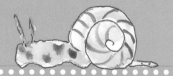

Photo of You in the World

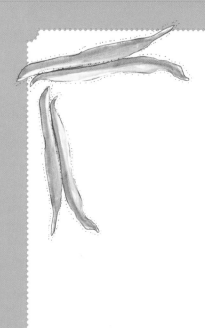

Place photo here.

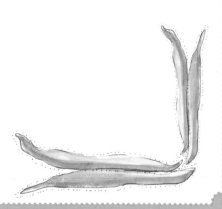

Your adventures are just beginning.

Where you went first: _____

_____

_____

_____

_____

_____.

What you did: _____

_____

_____

_____

_____

_____.

Who you were with: _____

_____

_____

_____

_____

_____

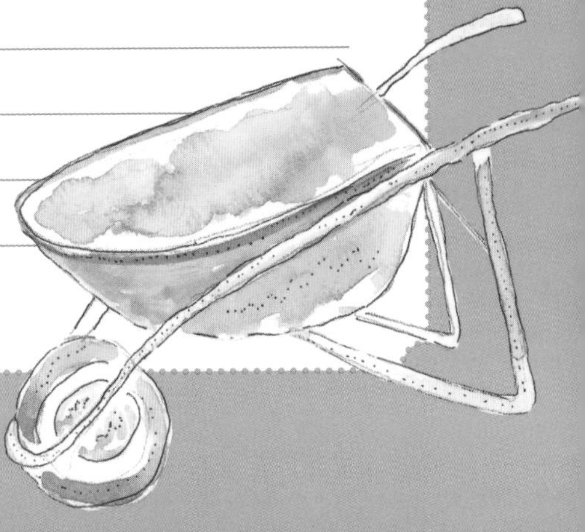

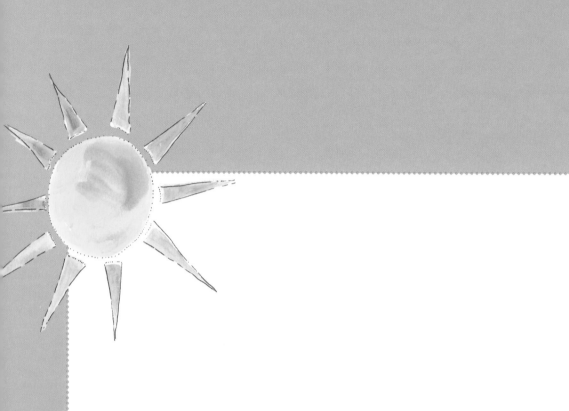

Place photo of baby having a good time here.

You are our little sunshine.

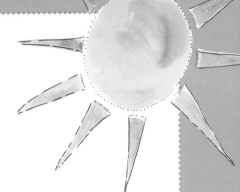

Place photo of baby's smile here.

You first smiled on _____
_____.
We were at _____
_____. We're pretty sure you smiled at
_____ first.

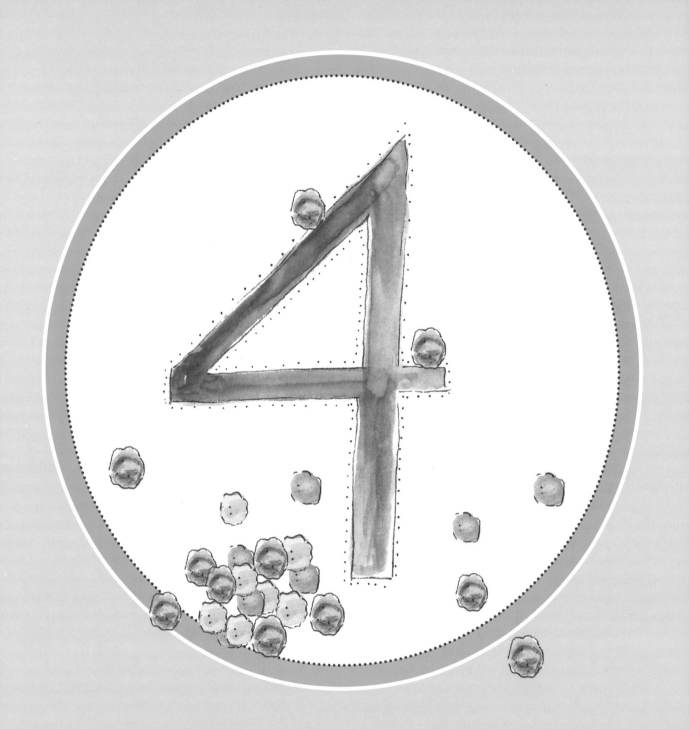

MONTHS

Look what you can do.

Place photo here.

Height: _____

Weight: _____

Thoughts about Month Four

_____

_____

_____

_____

_____

_____

_____

_____

_____

_____

_____

_____

_____

_____

_____

_____

_____

_____

_____

FOUR MONTHS

You laugh mostly at _____
_____
_____.

Your cheeks are simply _____
_____.

You are looking at everything, especially _____
_____.

Your daily life right now is _____
_____.

You have made our family so much _____
_____.

Your thoughts on tummy time are _____
_____.

What we don't want to forget about this month of your life is _____
_____
_____.

We couldn't be more happy / relieved / exhausted /
hungry / giddy / emotional / grateful.

(Circle what applies.)

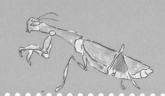

Your Nursery

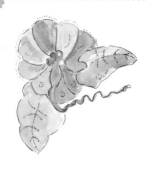

Place photo here.

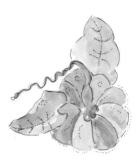

Something special about your room is _____

_____

_____

_____

_____

_____.

The theme/patterns/colors are _____

_____

_____

_____

_____

_____.

Your favorite thing in your room is _____

_____

_____

_____

_____

_____.

Our favorite thing about your room is _____

_____

_____

_____

_____

One word that describes your room best is _____

_____

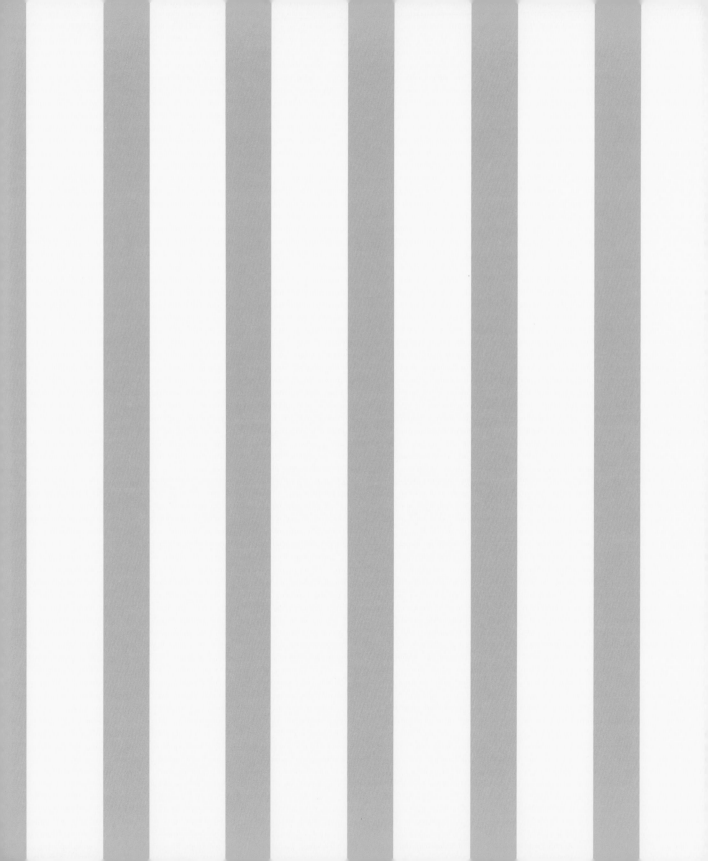

Checkups and Doctor Visits

Date	Weight/Height	Notes

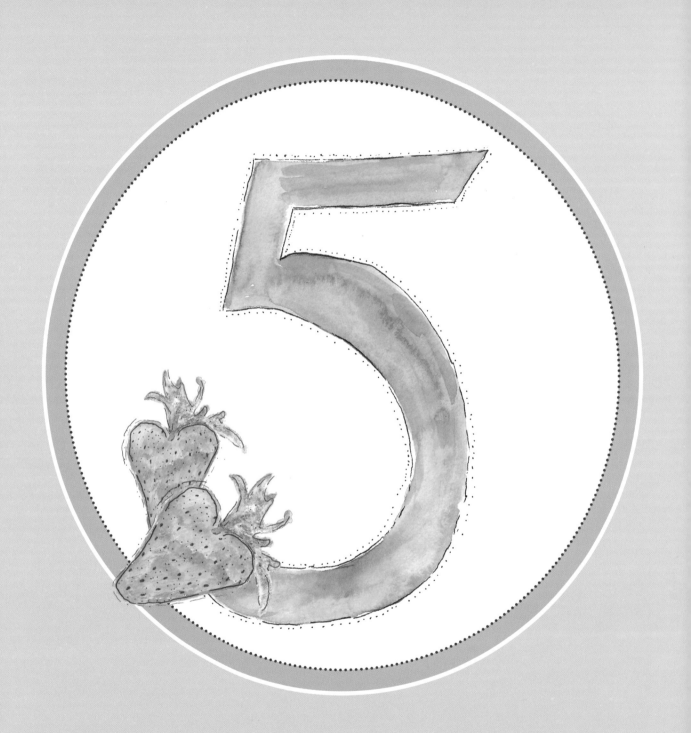

MONTHS

Look at that face.

Place photo here.

Height: _____

Weight: _____

Thoughts about Month Five

FIVE MONTHS

You can grab things now. What you grab most is _____

_____

_____.

You want to be on the go. Mostly you want to go _____

_____.

Your nap schedule these days is _____

_____.

How you get to sleep is _____

_____.

Something you just can't get enough of is _____

_____.

We sing _____

_____to you all the time. And play

_____.

What we don't want to forget about this month of your life is _____

_____.

We couldn't be more happy / relieved / exhausted /
hungry / giddy / emotional / grateful.

(Circle what applies.)

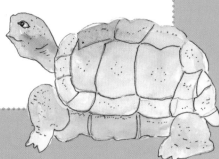

Place photo of happy times with baby here.

Baby's Vine of Happiness

Date: _____

How happy does it make baby?

Deliriously happy: ....

Happy: ....

Smiley: ....

Peachy: ....

Cranky: ....

Super cranky pants: ....

Fill in blanks with things that make baby happy (i.e., special toy, song, person, etc.). And what doesn't (shots, diaper changes, 5 p.m., etc.).

Baby, I want you to know...

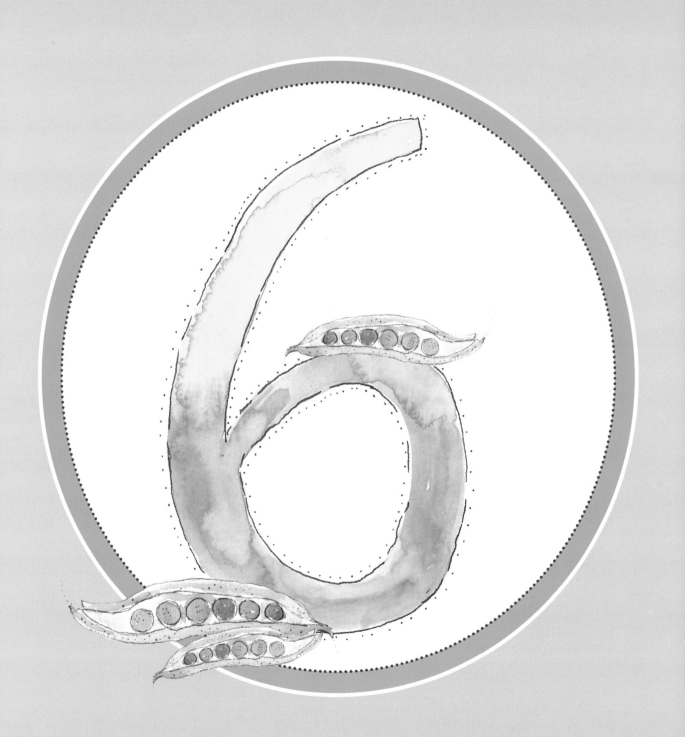

MONTHS

You are a sweet pea.

Place photo here.

Height: _____

Weight: _____

Thoughts about Month Six

SIX MONTHS

We can't believe you are halfway through your first year! These first six months have been _____ and also
_____.

What is helping us be better parents for you is _____
_____.

The way you like to get around is _____
_____.

They say your eye color is set now and it's a lovely _____.
When you wake in the morning, the first thing you want is _____
_____.

Our most special time together is _____
_____.

You have changed our life for the better especially by making us
_____
_____.

What we don't want to forget about this month of your life is _____
_____.

We couldn't be more happy / relieved / exhausted /
hungry / giddy / emotional / grateful.

(Circle what applies.)

Here's how you spent your first holidays, sweet one.

New Year's Eve

_____

_____

Valentine's Day

_____

_____

St. Patrick's Day

_____

_____

Easter/Passover

_____

_____

Fourth of July

_____

_____

Halloween

_____

_____

_____

Thanksgiving

_____

_____

_____

Christmas/Hanukkah/Kwanzaa

_____

_____

_____

Baptism/Christening

_____

_____

_____

Other special days for our family

_____

_____

_____

_____

_____

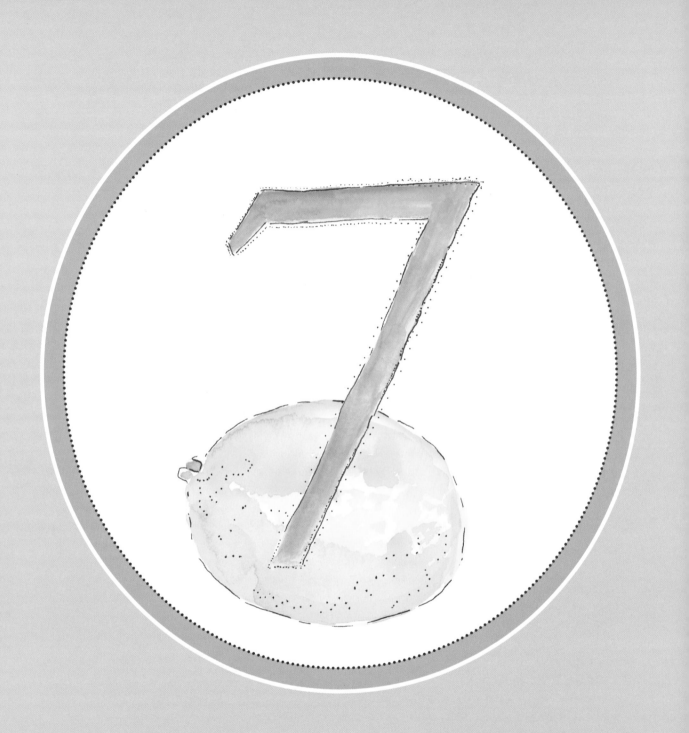

MONTHS

We can't get enough of you.

Place photo here.

Height: _____

Weight: _____

Thoughts about Month Seven

SEVEN MONTHS

You know that you definitely like _____ but not
_____.

When you meet a new person, you are _____
_____.

When we have to leave you for a bit, you _____
_____.

Your current bedtime routine includes _____
_____.

You are your happiest when _____
_____.

On the weekends, we _____
_____.

What's really special about you, baby, is _____
_____.

What we don't want to forget about this month of your life is _____
_____.

We couldn't be more happy / relieved / exhausted /
hungry / giddy / emotional / grateful.

(Circle what applies.)

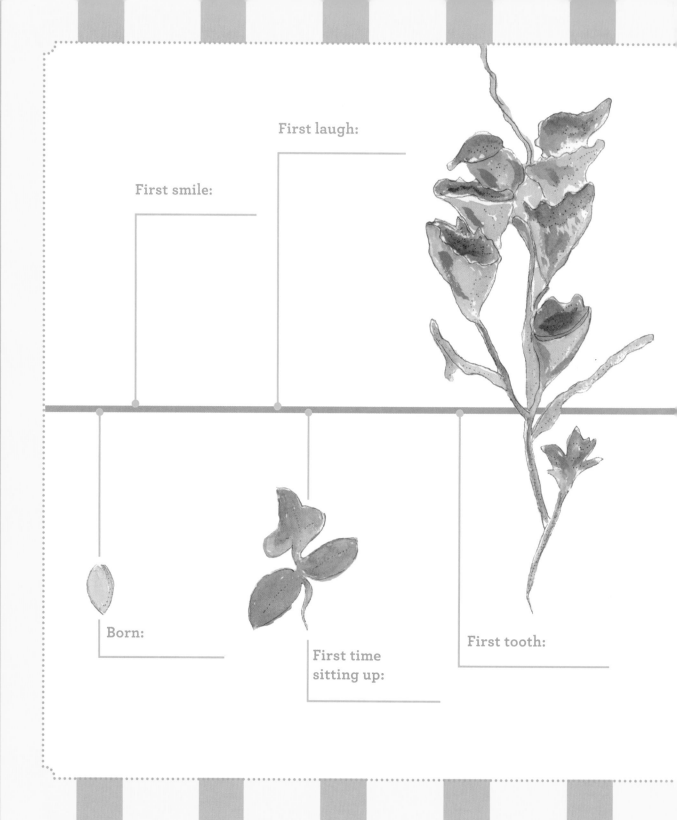

First laugh:

First smile:

Born:

First time
sitting up:

First tooth:

Timeline of Our
Little Pumpkin's Firsts

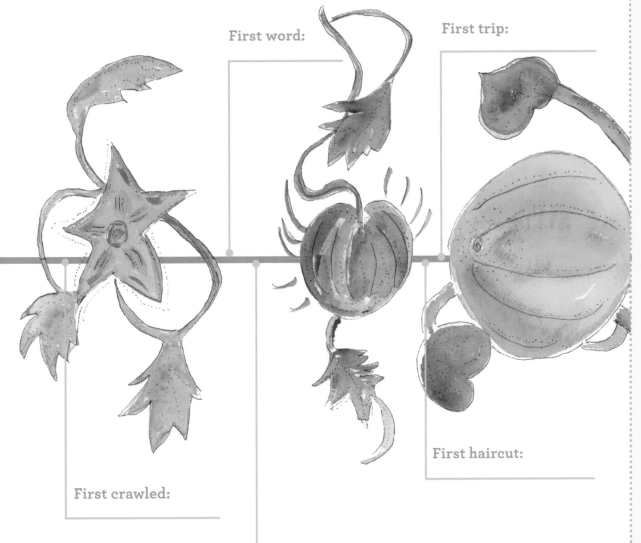

First word:

First trip:

First crawled:

First step:

First haircut:

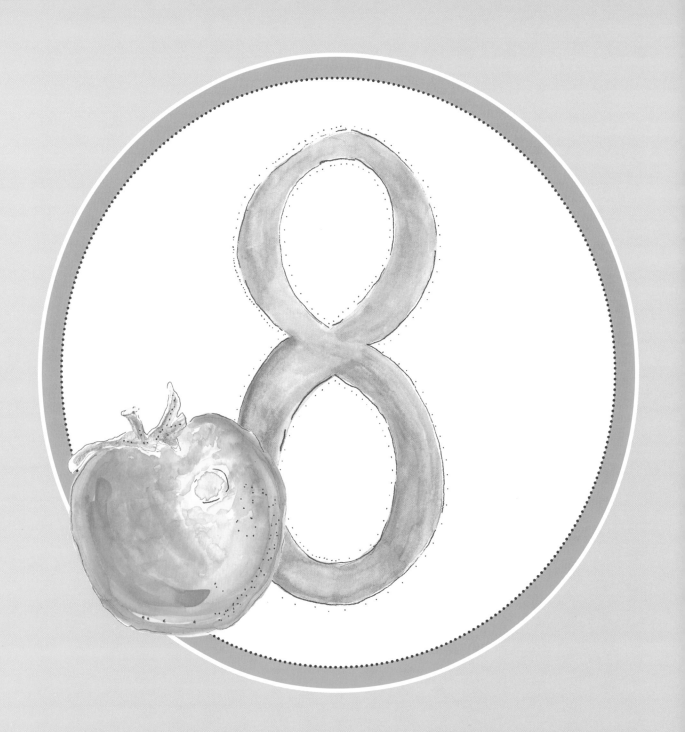

MONTHS

You are getting so big.

Place photo here.

Height: _____

Weight: _____

Thoughts about Month Eight

EIGHT MONTHS

You are really becoming your own person. We know this because

_____

_____.

Something I'm noticing about your personality that I hope stays

forever is your _____

_____.

Your hair is simply _____.

Nothing makes you happier than _____ or sadder than

_____

_____.

Your opinion on car rides: _____

_____.

Outside, you adore _____ the most.

You have already made us reevaluate our _____

_____.

What we don't want to forget about this month of your life is _____

_____.

We couldn't be more happy / relieved / exhausted /
hungry / giddy / emotional / grateful.

(Circle what applies.)

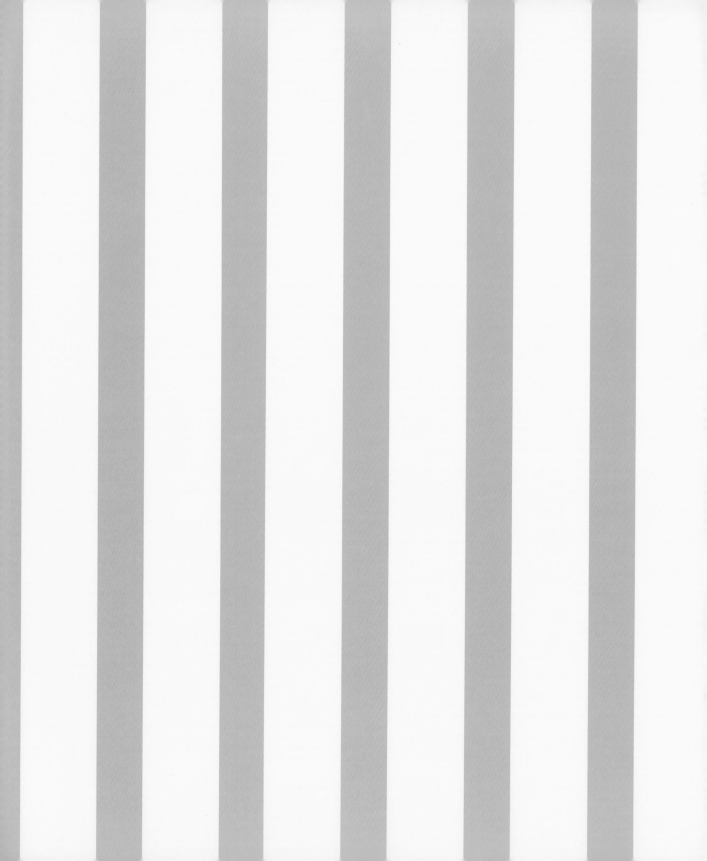

Pumpkin Pie Chart

Baby's day on: _____

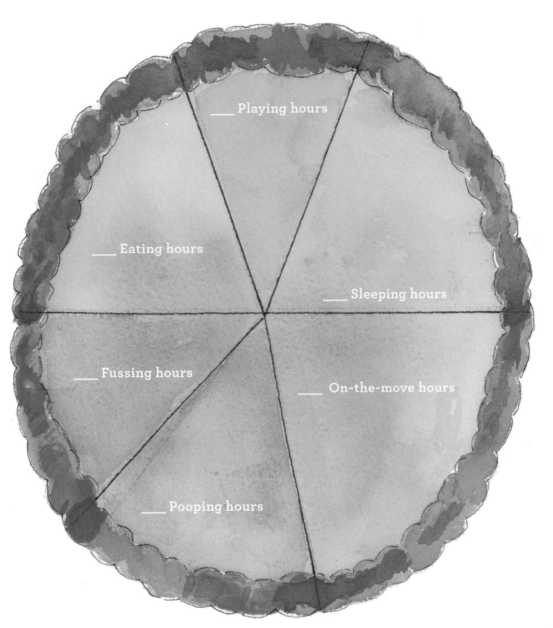

____ Playing hours

____ Eating hours

____ Sleeping hours

____ Fussing hours

____ On-the-move hours

____ Pooping hours

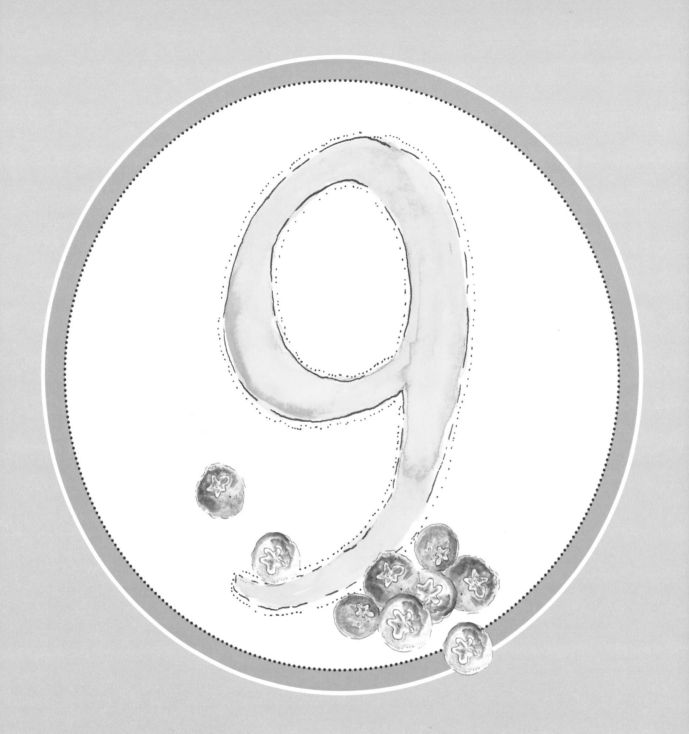

MONTHS

You are the berries.

Place photo here.

Height: _____

Weight: _____

Thoughts about Month Nine

NINE MONTHS

Your favorite way to spend an afternoon is _____
_____ .

The thing you do that cracks us up is _____
_____
_____ .

Our best family time is _____
_____ .

We couldn't be prouder of your _____
_____
_____ .

What frustrates you is _____
_____
_____ .

What we don't want to forget about this month of your life is _____
_____
_____
_____

We couldn't be more happy / relieved / exhausted /
hungry / giddy / emotional / grateful.

(Circle what applies.)

Baby's Faves

Lovie

_____

_____

Food

_____

_____

Pet

_____

_____

Thing to do

_____

_____

Friend

_____

_____

_____

_____

View

_____
_____
_____

Place

_____
_____
_____

Toy

_____
_____
_____

Song

_____
_____
_____

Game

_____
_____
_____
_____

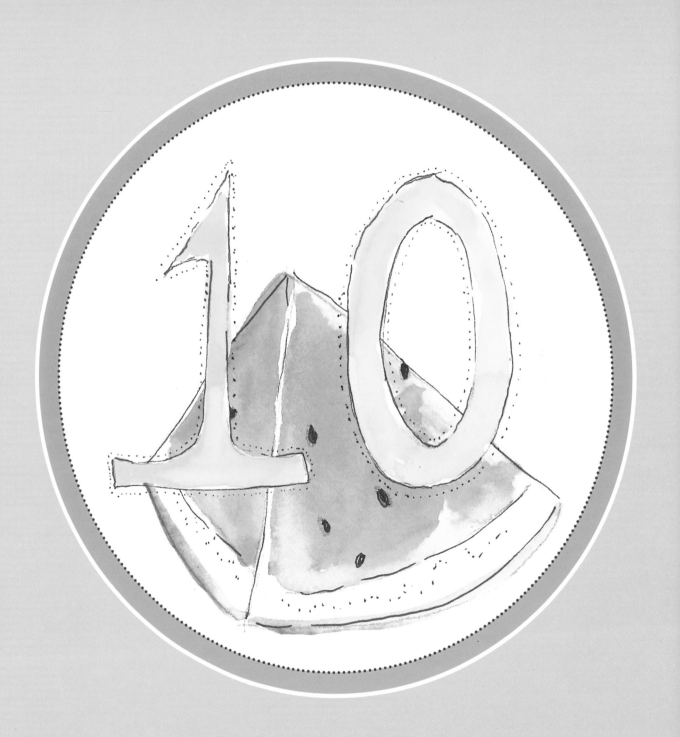

MONTHS

You are a perfect ten.

Place photo here.

Height: _____

Weight: _____

Thoughts about Month Ten

_____

_____

_____

_____

_____

_____

_____

_____

_____

_____

_____

_____

_____

_____

_____

_____

_____

_____

_____

_____

TEN MONTHS

Your temperament at the moment is _____
_____.

You are on the move and are usually headed to _____
_____.

Your feeling on new people is _____
_____.

The joy you have brought to our lives is _____
_____.

Your independence is making us _____
_____.

You are communicating and it sounds like this: _____
_____

and we think it means _____
_____.

What we don't want to forget about this month of your life is _____
_____
_____.

We couldn't be more happy / relieved / exhausted /
hungry / giddy / emotional / grateful.

(Circle what applies.)

Place photo of happy times with baby here.

Baby's Vine of Happiness

Date: _____

How happy does it make baby?

Deliriously happy: ....

Happy: ....

Smiley: ....

Peachy: ....

Cranky: ....

Super cranky pants: ....

Fill in blanks with things that make baby happy (i.e., special toy, song, person, etc.). And what doesn't (shots, diaper changes, 5 p.m., etc.).

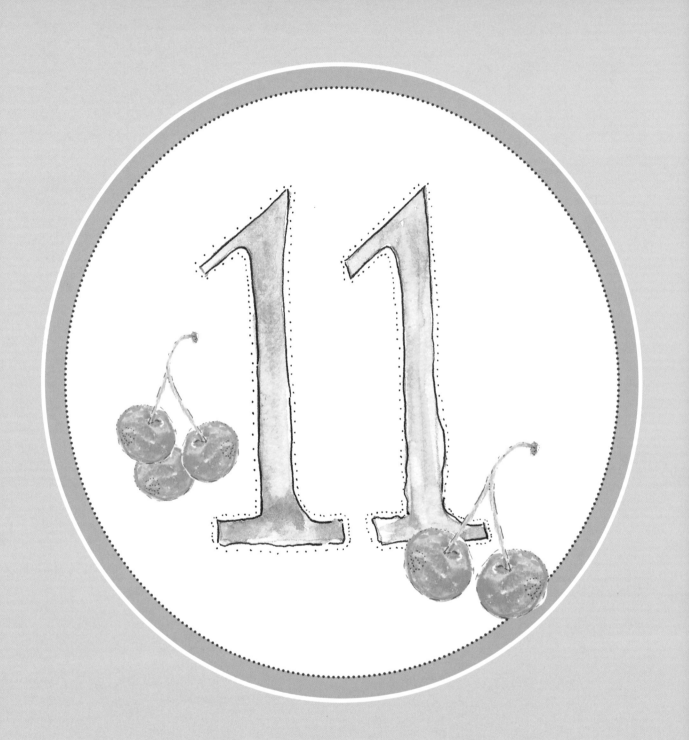

MONTHS

We love you bunches.

Place photo here.

Height: _____

Weight: _____

Thoughts about Month Eleven

ELEVEN MONTHS

You are most definitely saying things like _____
_____. We think it means
_____.

You love _____ more than anything.

Nap time these days is _____
_____.

At bedtime, you want _____
_____.

We know we are not perfect parents, but we are getting better at
_____
_____
_____. We are still working on
_____.

Baby, you have taught us so much about _____
_____.

What we don't want to forget about this month of your life is _____
_____.

We couldn't be more happy / relieved / exhausted /
hungry / giddy / emotional / grateful.

(Circle what applies.)

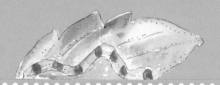

Photo of You in the World

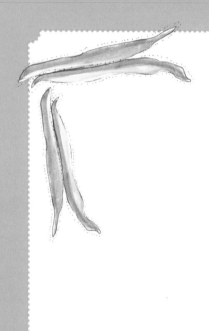

Place photo here.

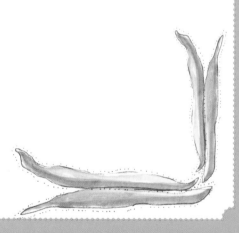

Your adventures have already begun.

You like to go _____

_____

_____ with

_____

_____

_____.

Your favorite way to travel is by _____

_____

_____.

We always bring _____

_____

_____.

Sometimes we _____

_____

_____

_____

_____

_____

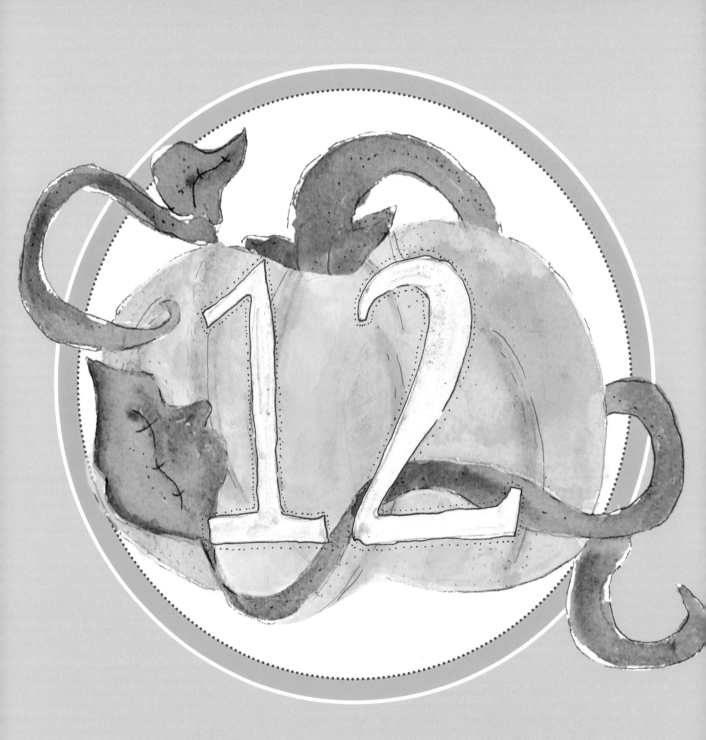

MONTHS

What a cute little pumpkin.

Place photo here.

Height: _____

Weight: _____

Thoughts about Month Twelve

TWELVE MONTHS

When we have to tell you "no," you usually react by _____

_____.

Your favorite word at the moment is _____

_____, and when you say it, you point to

_____

_____.

These days, you can _____

_____ all by yourself.

At mealtime, you usually prefer _____

_____.

Here's how you get around: _____

_____.

You have surprised us in so many ways. Mostly with your _____

_____.

What we don't want to forget about this month of your life is _____

_____

_____.

We couldn't be more happy / relieved / exhausted /
hungry / giddy / emotional / grateful.

(Circle what applies.)

Letter to You on Your
First Birthday

_____

_____

_____

_____

_____

_____

_____

_____

_____

_____

_____

_____

_____

_____

_____

_____

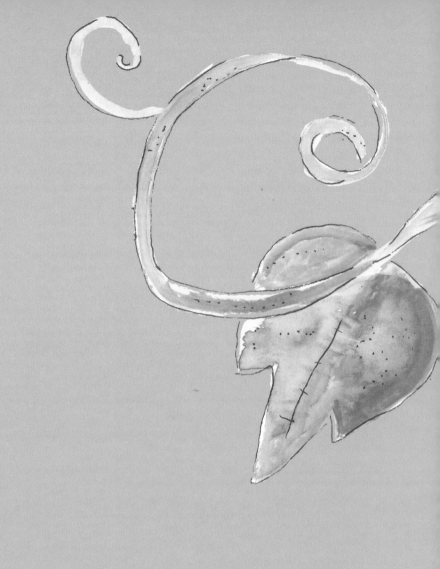

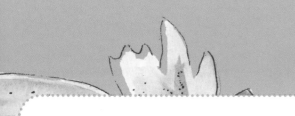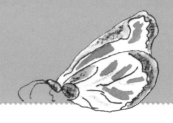

Share your baby's monthly photo with help from these sweet *From Pea to Pumpkin* signs. Simply cut out the appropriate page each month (look on both sides!) and place with baby for a photo. Go for whatever baby is up for: sleeping, sitting, drooling! Collect all twelve photos and make a share-worthy keepsake for your little one to treasure.

1

MONTH

PeatoPumpkin.com

2

MONTHS

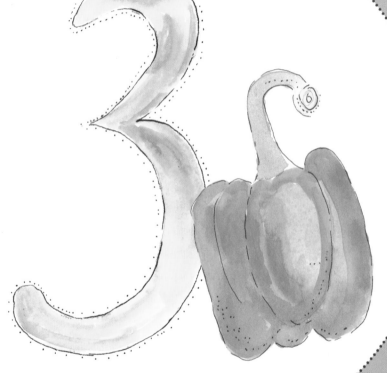

· PeatoPumpkin.com ·

MONTHS

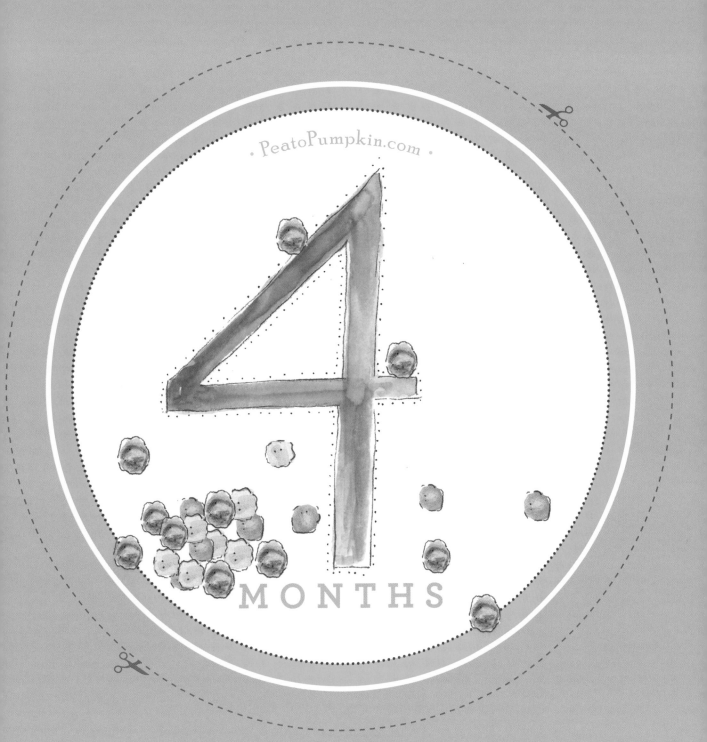

PeatoPumpkin.com

MONTHS

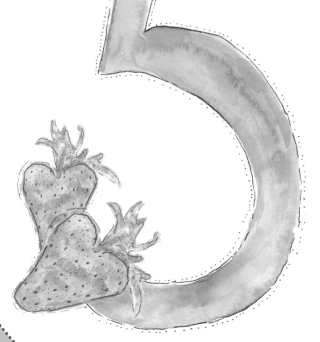

5

MONTHS

PeatoPumpkin.com

6

MONTHS

PeatoPumpkin.com

7

MONTHS

PeatoPumpkin.com

8

MONTHS

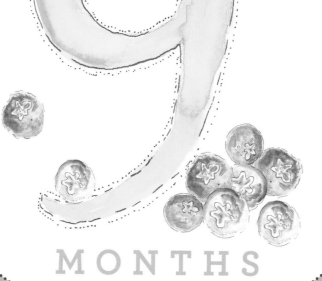

MONTHS

PeatoPumpkin.com

10

MONTHS

PeatoPumpkin.com

11

MONTHS

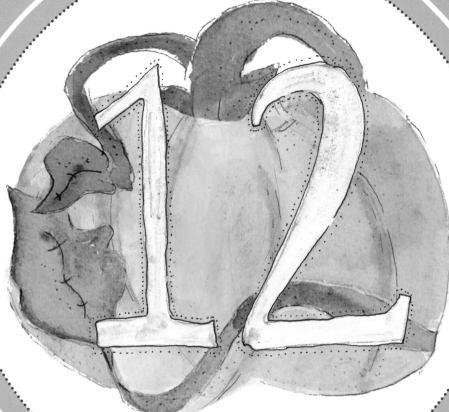

PeatoPumpkin.com

MONTHS

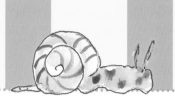

About the Author/ Illustrator

Geralyn Broder Murray is a writer of advertising, books, and other things that make people happy/buy stuff/do stuff. You can find her online at www.bigshotwriter.com.

For more on *From Pea to Pumpkin*, go to PeatoPumpkin.com. "Like" us on Facebook for regular P2P updates throughout your baby's first years and beyond.